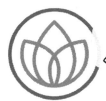

CONNECT
TO YOUR ONE

RUPA MEHTA
FOUNDER OF NALINIKIDS
& NALINI METHOD

CONNECT
TO YOUR ONE

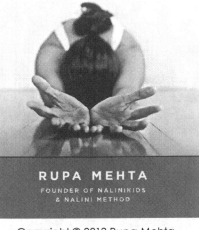

RUPA MEHTA
FOUNDER OF NALINIKIDS
& NALINI METHOD

ISBN: 1489521895
ISBN-13: 9781489521897

Head Editor: Amanda Madden
Copy Editor: Mackenzie Jessen

Acknowledgements

Thank you for picking up my book. I really hope it inspires you. It has served many roles for me, but most importantly, it is a letter to honor my parents. They deserve huge recognition for providing me with a safe, secure upbringing, unconditional love, freedom, support, and self-confidence. The reality my parents embody is undeniably delightful and impactful. Their usage of words has guided my life and shaped my identity. Thanks Mom and Dad.

I also want to recognize and thank all the dedicated and committed educators, individuals and students who have and continue to work endlessly to support NaliniKIDS. All of you are the heart of the NaliniKIDS mission and pump its vision.

Contents

A Letter to You · 1

Words Matter

The Weight of Words · 7
Connect to Your One · 13
Dad. Mom. · 17

Happiness

Dad · 25
"The solution is born before the problem." · · · · · · · · · · · · · · · 35
"No one can take away your happiness." · · · · · · · · · · · · · · · · 43
"Don't magnify successes or failures." · · · · · · · · · · · · · · · · · · 55

Balance

Mom · 65
"Shut up. Sit. Smile." · 75
"Love yourself dearly. Be yourself completely.
    Treat yourself occasionally." · 83
"Let go. Love. Live." · 91

Connect

"Say thank you." · 99

A Letter to You

Dear reader,

When I was younger, it felt naïve to speak of wanting to transform the world; I thought I was too small and the world was too big. But now, after years of growing my business, meeting countless inspirational individuals, and teaching well over 10,000 classes, I feel no matter what size I am or what reach I have, that it is my duty to try.

I named my business after my mom, Nalini Mehta, because I wanted to create an environment that emanated the feeling I had around her — a feeling of being accepted, encouraged, nurtured, and challenged. Through idealistic eyes, I thought that if others could experience even a little of what I was blessed with growing up that the world would be a better place. I want to be the change I'd like to see in the world and I hope to inspire others to be that change as well. I want to live and share the greatest life I can and I want others to live and share their greatest lives as well.

Connect To Your One: NaliniKIDS

Mahatma Gandhi's famous words, "My life is my message" is a quote I wish we could all live by. I believe we all have messages and to live our greatest lives, we must know and share that message. My life - my message - is NaliniKIDS and Nalini Method.

My vision for NaliniKIDS and Nalini Method is to create a community for people to connect to their lives. A community that enables youth and adults across the world to connect and develop their emotional and physical strength to pursue their dreams and live happy and productive lives.

Throughout both my personal and professional life, I have found that if we can connect to our greatest bodies, minds and hearts, then we all have messages to share that could collectively transform the world. Can you imagine a world where we all experience each other's greatest lives?

I believe it requires a healthy body, mind and heart to connect to your life. When you are physically healthy, you have the confidence and strength to clear your mind. With a clear mind, you have the drive and desire to fully understand and embrace your heart. Once you understand your heart's personal message - what drives you in life - you will invest your time and energy into sharing your personal message with the world.

It's rather simple: We have the tools to build the lives we want, be the change we want to see in the world, and share our unique messages.

I hope is that this book's message will help you find your message.

Thank you for reading,
Rupa Mehta

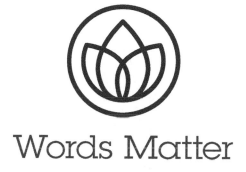

Words Matter

The Weight of Words

Do you think I'm fat? Do you think I'm ripped? Does this shirt make me look fat? I will get a great body if I just don't eat, right? What can I do to lose weight? I need to get this girl to like me, what should I do? Do you think if I lose weight, this boy will like me? What do you do to stay fit?

Those are the kinds of questions I am asked by thousands of students, young and old, who are fit, strong, flexible, and lean. I have been teaching adults since 2001 and kids since 2008. Six days a week I teach three to four group fitness classes to an affluent adult clientele on the Upper West Side of New York City and three days a week I teach school students, preK-12, from various backgrounds in Brooklyn and Manhattan.

Of course they ask me these questions; I am their fitness instructor and teacher. To some I'm their escape, their therapy, their routine, and to others, their reliable friend, their confidence, and their hope. Because I have come to develop a different definition of "weight," I believe many of my students—exercise enthusiasts, successful businessmen and women, fit and strong parents, nutritionists, dietians, public and private school students, physical education teachers and other popular health advocates—are so much more "overweight" than they could even imagine.

Physically fit and yet overweight? Yes. Our society's idea of weight is unbalanced. With an obsessive focus on only physical weight and disregard for a person's entire well-being, even the most popular fitness books, products, and services do a disservice to a captive audience looking not only to be healthier physically but also to feel great and be confident in their lives.

Having been asked these questions for years, I feel compelled to approach them in this book from a unique perspective. To truly transform and connect to our lives, we must rethink weight. The kind of weight loss that I know would benefit adults and kids looking to live their greatest lives requires something besides physical exercise and diet.

But, before we get into my message, let's look at the definition of *weight*.

> **Weight:** 1) a body's relative mass or the quantity of matter contained by it.
>
> 2) the heaviness of a person or thing.

This definition intrigues me—pounds are not even mentioned! In fact, weight is not about the scale; that's our society's interpretation. The bottom line is, you can be very fit and still be heavy.

Emotional weight can be just as alarming and detrimental as unhealthy physical weight. And, I see so many slim clients and students daily that look so heavy. Yes, they are in shape but their attitudes and behavior makes it seem like they have packed on an additional hundred pounds! This is an observation that needs to surface, be recognized, and dealt with.

After all, there is no perfect body, no perfect mind, and no perfect person. There is only the perfect you. Maybe you like to be full-figured or maybe you like to be thin—none of it matters if your spirit is weighed down. Rather than chase after the subjective notions of body and mind prescribed to us, why not trim down our ideals and discover our light, beautiful, and individual spirits?

A healthy person isn't weighed down by emotions. Instead, their true spirit shines so clear and vibrantly that the world can't help but experience it.

And, how we understand, articulate, and share our spirits with the world occurs through words. Let's say I wake up in the morning and tell myself, "I have to have a good day and be positive," or "I will only be happy when I lose weight," or "I'm so beautiful, nothing can bring me down." Before I even eat my breakfast, I've already started packing on the *weight of words*. Over the years, we have all accumulated this emotional weight, the *weight of words*, and just like we should be aware of what we eat, we should also be aware of the exact words we digest into our spirits. One word has the power to weigh much more than a single scoop of ice cream.

If we want to be healthy, fit and confident in our lives, we must learn to appreciate the *weight of words*. We will all experience the ultimate transformation only when we start to recognize and lose this emotional weight. And, it requires strength and conviction to challenge the ideas of pounds, food, exercise and perfection that intermingle so seamlessly in our society.

For most of us, going for a run outside for 30 minutes is much easier than devoting 30 minutes to a phone call to our mom and owning up to the words we said to her in a fight. It requires clarity and drive to reflect on our emotional weight; and, patience and accountability to understand the impact of the words we live with and by. If you can start to lose the *weight of words*, you will lose emotional weight and be on a loving, long-lasting path to a healthy spirit.

Going on the latest diet will not necessarily help us lose physical weight, but a desire to take ownership of our lifestyle will. Similarly, going to therapy or practicing yoga and meditation can help us in many ways, but won't be as effective if we don't take ownership of the words we use, have been exposed to, listen to, admire, and plan to live by.

Nalini is a word I live by. I named both *NaliniKIDS and Nalini Method* after my mom, Nalini Pinak Mehta.

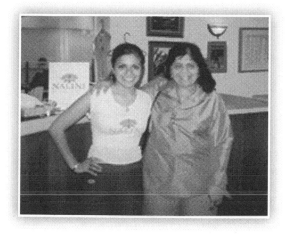

Nalini means *lotus*. The lotus flower starts small, growing from the bottom of a pond, bounded by mud and muck. As it slowly rises towards the water's surface, continually moving towards the light, it remains extraordinarily unsoiled despite the surrounding impurities. Once it comes to the surface of the water, the lotus bud begins to blossom and turns into a beautiful flower. Within Hinduism and Buddhism the lotus flower is a symbol for awakening to the spiritual reality of life.

For me, the spiritual reality of life involves awakening our spirits to the words we use and live by. Figuring out these words, realizing the power they can have on our lives, and embracing our ability to control our interpretations of them can drive us towards our spiritual light and lightness. Awakening ourselves to the *weight of words* will lead to a healthier spirit which will naturally give way to looking better, feeling better, and living a better life.

Connect to Your One

If your spirit were represented by one word, what would it be?

Now that I've posed the question, are you tempted to choose one immediately? But there are so many words, how do you know which one is yours? Is there a right or wrong answer? Can you really imagine having only one word to define and drive your life?

Think about it, just for a moment, all of the words you live with and by. It's comforting yet daunting to think of all the words we have been exposed to in our lives and even more overwhelming to think of choosing only one for our spirit.

Imagine having one word to guide your moral compass, your actions, your inner peace, and your resolve. I have already proposed that if your spirit is healthy, you have lost the *weight of words*. I want to take it one step further and state that if you can connect to your one word, and live your one word to the fullest, you will live your greatest life.

Let's look at the definition of spirit:

> **Spirit:** the vital principle of a person; the non-phys-
> ical part of a person, the soul, regarded as
> a person's true self.

Is YOUR true self reading this book? Does your true self hang out with your friends? Are you your true self at home? Is your true self talking to your mom/guardian over the phone? Does your true self introduce itself to new people? Does your true self wake up every morning? Do people know your true self? Do you know your true self?

If you can define your true self in one word and are able to live your word truthfully in all aspects of your life, then you will feel strong and healthy.

Due to its non-physical nature, it's not easy to come up with an objective evaluation of the state of your spirit. I mean where can you jump on a spirit scale? And, what would you even weigh?

You can use your one word to measure the weight of your spirit. Just as you cannot have multiple bodies and minds, by definition, your spirit cannot have multiple truths. And because we articulate and understand truths through words, your spirit cannot have multiple words to live by. If your spirit has too many truths or words to live by, it will be weighed down. If your spirit did not have a truth, it would not exist. You must know your one truth, your one word, to have a healthy, vibrant spirit.

If your spirit is weak and weighed down, your one word is being outbalanced by the weight of other words. If your spirit is strong and lifted up, you are living your one word and have lost the *weight of words*.

So, put this metric around your spirit. Test it now. Do you know your one word? Are you living your one word? If you jumped on the spirit scale, what would it say?

We have so many methods of measuring our physical weight and none to measure our emotional weight. We must create and abide by some type of emotional/spiritual measurement if we truly want to live healthier and happier lives. Once we discover our one word we can use it as a tool to assess the health of all aspects of your life.

Your spirit, your truth, has limitless potential-it is the one word that can drive you to live your greatest life. Connecting to your one word will not only let you create the life you want but it will allow the world to fully experience your life, your spirit, your truth - your message.

With so many words to choose from and the complexity of life, it is hard to choose just one word, so take your time. Although your past and future help to manifest your one word, it's not looking back or looking forward that will fully bring you to your truth; it's looking within that will connect you to your one.

The path to choosing your one word requires acknowledging the *weight of words* and asking yourself some tough questions.

Listening to your thoughtful answers will bring clarity. With that clarity you will have the motivation to trim all the words of your life into one word.

Starting a word detox, losing emotional weight and connecting to your one is the healthiest and best gift you can give yourself and the world. This is my journey to my one word.

Dad. Mom.

My dad sneezes in a way that makes me cringe—I mean, why won't he cover his mouth? My dad's obsession with following GPS makes me want to get lost and have no signal for hours just to prove a point. His overt confidence embarrasses me at times. His enthusiasm and fearlessness inspire me. I wonder how my mom makes it through the day when my dad won't shut up about his excitement about a new project. God, I am so much like him! But, it does seem like my mom has a lot to say, too, why else would she call me so much? Why doesn't she come to visit me more often, don't all Indian moms usually jump at the chance to do that? I hope to be even half the mom she is to me. I miss living near them. Why does more than two weeks with them make me so sleepy? I get tears in my eyes when I see my mom walk more slowly because of joint pain. Is she disappointed that I'm not married yet? I feel lucky that they always accept my choices. I want them to be a huge part of my future children's lives. Do they sit up at night and wonder about my future? Do they know that I don't mean to be defensive, but that I just can't help it sometimes? Do they know I talk about them all the time? Do they know how much I love them?

Dad. Mom. Just the mere words conjure up so many emotions for me. I mean, there they were in the beginning, the very beginning—from my cell development up to now. With or with-out my knowledge or invitation, physically or emotionally there or not, they've always been on my life journey.

It could be that you agreed with your parents' words and actions from the day you were born. Mmmm—probably not. Almost al-ways, to learn from our parents takes experience, time, distance, and even rebellion. As a first-generation Indian American, growing up with my parents' views wasn't always easy nor did the value in their lessons come naturally. For me, the value has grown out of my deep reflection upon their words, ideas, and actions. It's not about agreeing or disagreeing with my parents and their lessons and words; the immense value lies in the mere contemplation.

Whether you define yourself as fat or skinny, daughter or mother, guardian or father, young or old, gay or straight, adopted or biological, orphaned or parented, we all have the role of child. And, that is why I offer this book to everyone, all children, who could be more aware of the many worthwhile lessons they received in order to live a more resolved life. It is for children who admire their parents and their upbringing but haven't taken the time to fully understand why; children who have become too stubborn, self-absorbed, lazy, or entitled to fully appreciate their parents; children who have experienced vari-ous degrees of absenteeism, abandonment and loss; children who seek recovery from their childhood to feel that they can fully develop an identity, and current or future parents, once children, thinking about how they will raise their own.

I didn't have the desire to write this book at the age of 16, 20, or 25. Now, at 30, I feel that I have hit a milestone in maturity that has brought with it a refreshing and powerful perspective. When I look back, I feel an overwhelming sense of appreciation for living such a lucky, loved life. I feel that with one breath I could conquer the world and in that same breath accept my own death. I don't believe my successes have been earth-shattering, that I've accomplished everything I'd like to, or that I've enjoyed my friends and family to the fullest; I do have concrete goals, love to experience new things, and desire to spend more time with so many people. But, although I enjoy life, I know that if I died today, it would be with the knowledge that I have lived a good life, fulfilled my life's mission, and my spirit has shone. I believe this state of mind is the result of my upbringing—a gift from my parents.

I feel like our culture could use a reality check. We need less "my parents didn't do this" and more "thankfully, my parents did do this." Currently, accusations are much more prevalent. We tend to associate our parents only with our "bad" characteristics, our struggles and fears, and there is hardly any acknowledgment given to our parents regarding our "good" characteristics—our successes and accomplishments. Even the seemingly simple idea that they provided experiences that serve as a foundation gets forgotten. Acknowledgement seems to come only when prompted by some external force such as illness, a holiday, or a major life change. Bottom line: The words *dad* and *mom* carry a lot of weight. Why not lose some of the weight and see your parents in a different light, as simply a significant part of your life and foundation?

Whether our parents provided a shack or a mansion for us to grow up in, offered us harsh or kind words, they are our foundation. Personally, I was fortunate enough to experience a modest upbringing in Fairfax, Virginia, a college education, and a supported career path of teaching fitness to an affluent clientele. Throughout, many fortunate and privileged children, like myself, have surrounded me. So many of us seem to take for granted our blessed circumstances. But, if I think upon my own life and my parents' journey to America, I have been taught to see our problems as a liberty and luxury. We're lucky to have the computer that keeps freezing; the homework that makes us miss our favorite show; the caregiver that calls us early in the morning; and the saying from our father figure that we say to ourselves when we're feeling down. Realizing the numerous unrecognized gifts that we have can help us see our struggles in a different light. Instead of being frustrated with our peers, teachers, friends, siblings, or parents, we will be thankful for our education in life, relationships, family—our foundation. If we can accept and appreciate our foundation, whether it was ideal or not, broken or unbroken, we have the mental space and freedom to create our own truth.

As a result of my own reflection, I feel inspired to give thanks to all parents and caregivers who intentionally (and unintentionally) share life lessons with their children. As a thankful and loved person and hopefully a future parent myself, I hope that sharing the lessons of my life will motivate you to ask yourself an imperative question on the path to connecting to your one word: "How do the words of your parents or guardians influence you?"

My home is built on the meshing of two worlds, Indian and American. Given that English is my parents' second language, they have a different perspective on the meaning of words. As a result, they make an intense effort to understand the English words they use in order to be accurate in their speech. As you read this book, you will see that their perspective on words has transformed into a unique view of the world. I once asked my parents to define life in one word. My dad quickly said, "happiness", and my mom immediately after said, "balance". As you explore my parents' life lessons, I think you will see how appropriate to their lives each of their words are. Everything my dad says and does embodies happiness and my mom's words and actions embody balance. In my life, one thing has become very clear to me—the way you live and want to live your life will inevitably be reflected in everything you say and do, so you have to embrace and choose your words wisely. My parents' personalities, upbringing, experiences, and goals led them each to their word. Knowing and embracing the one word that reflects their spirits and drives their lives allows them to not be weighed down. And when I reflect on my life lessons, experiences, and hopes for the future, and trim down the words that surround me into one, the word I choose to define and drive my life is—connect.

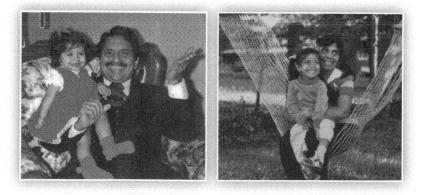

Throughout our lives, the people who raised us expose us to words that inevitably influence us. While reading this book, I hope you will think of their words, the words you currently use, and the words that bear the most *weight* in your life. Our spirits will begin to experience lightness when we take the time to realize how words work for us and against us. And, we will revel in ultimate health, true freedom, and potential when we embrace our ability to decide.

I want to share with you the weight of the words behind my life lessons and inspire you to articulate and interpret the life lessons taught to you by your parents or guardians. Understanding my life lessons by reflecting on the words I grew up with has allowed me to realize my one word.

Ultimately, accepting my parents' impact on my journey has given me the ability to consciously and confidently create my own life lessons and live and share my spirit - my one word.

Connect to Your One is the process of acknowledging the *weight of words*, self-reflection, and acceptance of the lessons you have learned in your life.

It may sound scary to reflect and transform your spirit into only one word, but losing the weight of having to define your life through all the various, subjective standards the world offers could be the most liberating path you could ever take.

As you read the following pages, keep the concept of the *weight of words* in the back of your mind. Consider this new process. Reflect on your life and think about the words that surround you, the control you have in interpreting them, and what it means to tap into or discover one word to guide your path.

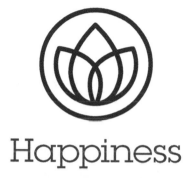

Happiness

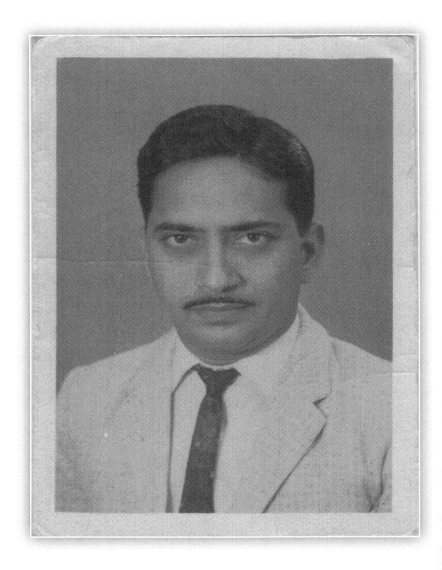

Dad

Although he is seventy years old, my dad, Pinak Ambalal Mehta, has the vivid imagination, mood swings, contagious enthusiasm, overflowing love, relentless motor-mouth capability, and stubbornness of a seven-year-old.

My dad was born in a railroad boxcar (a covered freight wagon) in India and has been on the move ever since. Because my grandfather was a railroad train master, my dad moved every three years, attending 29 schools in his lifetime. Due to the nature of his father's work and a large family (he was the second youngest of nine children), he grew up very poor. His family lived near the railroad tracks in the jungles of India in isolated environments, enclosed in nature with no running water, sleeping under trees. He watched his father manage the station, load goods, and ward off gangs of thieves. Once, he even witnessed his father being brutally beaten by more than 30 robbers.

How does a man from the jungles of India come to the US and become one of the first Indian American lawyers successfully practicing in Washington D.C.? Pure self-confidence and determination.

My dad is a strong-willed, highly optimistic man. With his unwavering strength of mind, he educated himself, moved out of his poor upbringing, and came to America with $8 in his pocket. He became a lawyer, started several small businesses including a printing company, a hotel, a liquor store, and a highly reputable heating and air-conditioning business and put two kids through undergraduate and graduate school.

My dad defines life on his own terms; he thinks anything is possible. Beyond money, fame, family and education, he still believes much more is possible. Even when what he sets out to do doesn't happen within six months, a year, or even longer, he has faith it will. More importantly, if something doesn't happen at all, he isn't affected; he relishes the journey. He's a go-getter who isn't attached to the "getting." He likes the spirit of life, projects, ventures, ideas, and goals and is not attached to the outcomes.

His unique character and youthful spiritedness has allowed him to openly and excitedly adapt to America; he always encourages himself and our family to try new things. He pushed my mom to learn to drive in the US, to travel alone, and to make a career for herself—all uncommon for a traditional Indian woman. He encouraged me to travel overseas by myself for three months when I was 14 and cheered me on when I quit my well-paid job to become an entrepreneur at 23.

As adamant as he is about his family trying new things, he's even more passionate about capturing and documenting his family's complete life experiences. At any given activity—dinner, birthday, family trip, or first day at a new job—you can find my dad in his 1981 Reebok classics and K-mart T-shirt with a $3,000 video camera and $1,000 camera carefully wrapped around his neck like gold medals on an Olympian. My dad will spend any amount of money on things that perpetuate family time and building a legacy. He preaches that igniting memories through film and photos is worth more than any material item. He once bought a new couch and videotaped my mom and him saying good-bye to the old couch we had for fifteen years! All in all, we have 176 neatly labeled videotapes, 22 8mm silent films, and thousands of pictures of family, friends, and memorable moments.

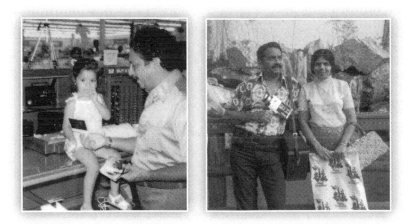

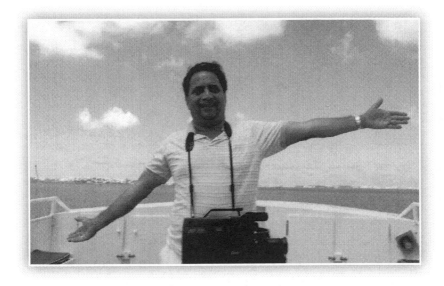

From buying a new couch to his children learning to drive, my dad can take any moment, circumstance, place, or object and make it larger than life and infuse it with happiness.

Everything from his videos to his home represents his loving demeanor, capability to create, and desire to share with others. Because of his huge personality, my family home, which my dad calls "heaven on earth," is always filled with a powerful joy of life.

If you entered my beloved house, American grandness and Indian spirituality would wonderfully charge your eyes. My home is not a random assembly of things, but a personal, loving time capsule of my dad's Indian roots, admiration of technology, affinity with nature, interest in American capitalism and opportunity, and love for his family—it truly is his "heaven on earth."

The most sacred place in my home is the pooja (Indian word for prayer) room which embodies both the Hindu and Jain religions. And, just like all the other rooms in my home, it has the special Pinak touch. It is a space filled with mismatched furniture, color, and meaningful objects that somehow all magically harmonize. Christmas lights, sandalwood chairs, colorfully framed photos of my grandparents and religious figures, and spiritual gifts from friends of all religions live in the ever-evolving pooja room. Everything in the room symbolizes something important, precious, and divine, even the wallpaper. My dad continues to keep the childish sailboat wallpaper left there from the previous owners because he says it represents "the ups and downs and peaceful ocean ride of life." My parents find complete peace and appreciation for life in the pooja room, praying and listening to Indian folk songs every morning and evening.

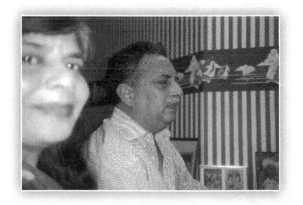

My dad doesn't just collect stuff; he generously and unpredictably gathers gifts for his home that inevitably take on his personality and reflect his jovial energy. For example, in the middle of our dining room is a grand hand-carved, gold-leafed wooden swing from India that my dad bought because he was in awe of its artistic beauty. But, rather than simply admire it, he made it a part of his life. He and my mom sit there and talk, sharing fresh coconut juice on the weekends. I also admire that my dad can just as enthusiastically find equal beauty in less artistic things, for example, a glow-in-the dark plastic tree sculpture that is the centerpiece of our wine bar.

And because he easily finds distinction and beauty in objects and people and showers his family with that loving attitude, my whole family truly appreciates the swing and the sculpture; his spirited love is simply contagious. It's because of this quality that my mom, who had always been terrified of water, learned to swim at the age of 60. My dad takes such infectious pride in our pool that my mom was able to not only try something new, but also to overcome a fear. My dad is so proud of my mom's efforts that he works hard to create a pool atmosphere that my mom enjoys and is comfortable in. Close to 10 water floaties, five foam boards, 20 water weights, and five pairs of goggles are all within arm's reach for her.

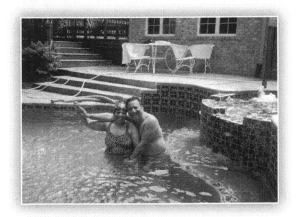

I have yet to meet another 70-year-old man who approaches life with more youthful enthusiasm than my dad. His hobbies and interests are endless. A 100-inch projector and a 60-inch flat screen TV sit side by side in his living room; two top-of-the-line computers and two of the latest iPads installed with every program imaginable live in the library, which is also filled with memoirs of American presidents and business tycoons; and four gold-plated small Indian copper cups that my dad passion-ately drinks out of every morning for "good luck" and "vitamin benefits" are positioned safely on the kitchen counter. Every inch of my home embodies my dad's character, his awe of life, and most importantly, family.

Family comes first for my dad. He is forever trying to create an even better life for us by thinking about, encouraging, and help-ing us enjoy our lives. He talks to me any time of the night, sends me personalized, computer-made cards every birthday, offers fatherly advice generously—and not only to me but also to all of my friends—and he'll cut up mangoes for anyone in his home with so much love and excitement, they actually taste sweeter. The love he has for me extends to those close to me; he has met all my friends and knows all of their phone numbers in case there is an emergency. He is interested in the details of my life and treats me as a person, independent of him, with my own identity.

His encouragement of me to live in the moment and define how I feel has helped me gain self-awareness. For example, when I was 12, he videotaped me before and after I got my braces, asking me how I felt, how the procedure went, how I was going to care for them, what I expected to get out of them, and told me to say hello to my family in India. My dad's deep interest and involvement in my life, while difficult to tolerate at times, has built my self-confidence. He works hard to understand my goals and pushes me to achieve them. He is the person who pushed me to ask for a raise after one month of working and to learn how to change the oil in my new car. He forces me to stay up-to-date on important and even non-important world affairs; I get up to eight emails a day from him ranging from a touching article about a tsunami survivor to a funny YouTube video about Beyoncé. Most importantly, he accepts, follows, and inspires my dreams.

If my dad could, he would share his heart and home with everyone. And if you were a guest in my home, the first thing you would see is his big smile, complete with the endearing gap between his two front teeth, which he claims is for good luck. The infectious smile emanating from this five-foot-six man would capture all of your attention. My mom would then hurry to greet you from the kitchen with some homemade Indian treats and my dad would grab his camera to capture this moment.

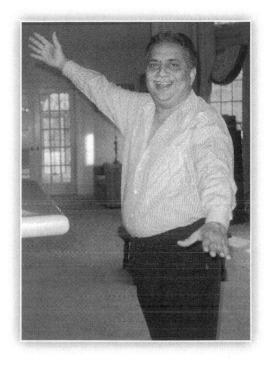

"The solution is born before the problem."

What if I told you that the world was filled with solutions but no problems? You might think I was idealistic, unaware, and unrealistic—exactly what I thought about my dad when I was growing up. You failed a test? Not a problem. You broke your leg? Not a problem. You have a deadly virus? Not a problem. As a kid, I was dumbfounded. How were these not legitimate problems? They felt like problems and everyone around me, from friends to doctors, also defined them that way.

My dad's favorite saying has always been "The solution is born before the problem." I heard it nearly every day growing up, and when I finally understood the power it has to transform one's perspective on life, it became my favorite saying, too.

When I heard this saying as a child, it didn't make sense. Is it even possible for the solution to exist before the problem? In fact, it is. It doesn't seem natural to us because our culture promotes the validity of problems coming first. We are inclined to see a problem first and look for solutions later. This lesson was the most difficult for me to understand because it required a mind shift that didn't feel natural but with time and experience, it became clear to me. Whether the lesson feels natural to you the first time or not, I think it's beneficial to be open and patient and stay with it.

Let's begin with the dictionary definitions of *solution* and *problem*.

> **Solution**: a means of solving a problem or dealing with a difficult situation.

> **Problem**: a matter or situation regarded as unwelcome or harmful and needing to be dealt with and overcome.

Here, the negativity of a problem is emphasized and a solution is only considered in terms of the problem. Growing up, I was taught that thinking of a problem as a "matter or situation that is unwelcome or harmful" is limiting and distracting. By focusing on the negativity of the problem, we attach ourselves to "fixing" the problem rather than finding a solution.

When you emotionally allow your problem to outweigh your search for a solution, you aren't as open to the many options that are possible solutions. In fact, both solutions and problems are just options, one that works and one that doesn't. Consider the following alternative definitions.

> **Solution:** An _option_ that causes a desired result at a desired time.

> **Problem:** A _solution_ that doesn't cause a desired result at a desired time.

This lesson is about seeing problems alternately, as solutions that are simply not functioning as such. To simplify, think of problems and solutions in terms of trying on shoes. If one doesn't fit (problem), you try on other shoes (options) until one does fit (solution).

Before writing this book, I had been looking for something to fill my time and add new meaning to my life, particularly regarding my business. As I mentioned earlier, I have operated my own fitness studio and taught classes six days a week for the past seven years. Although exhausting, it's my baby and I love it. I started the business at the age of 23 and have dedicated my life to building the business one client at a time. From teaching one client a day and begging people to spread the word to having close to 1,000 clients a month, prominent press coverage, and celebrity clientele, it has successfully grown over the years. But, although I have seen steady growth, I have lost some motivation and am close to my capacity in terms of teachers and space. To develop further, I would have to let my "baby" grow up and expand outside of my studio's walls and hire more teachers.

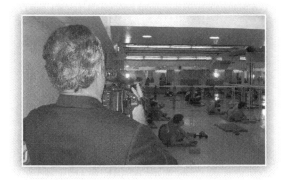

My first idea was to approach one of the country's most reputable fitness companies about buying my business. I confidently, yet nervously, wrote to the CEO of the company, and he wrote back the same day! The following week, representatives of the company came to take my class and see the studio. I was reveling in energy and enthusiasm as we met and talked about what a potential partnership could look like. Although nothing was solidified, the possibility was bringing an excitement to my days and giving me something to work on and look forward to; I had successfully filled my time and added new meaning to my life.

As I was daydreaming about a buy-out, in reality things were slowing down. I wrote a follow-up email to the company's representatives and did not receive a response. I waited and waited, and when they contacted me two months later, I was both shocked and relieved. They brought more people to the studio. Once again, there was momentum. We met and fully discussed the possibility of partnering as well as building a custom space in their new large facility, which was set to open in three months. They said I could expect a formal proposal in two weeks and the final transaction in four. I left the meeting on cloud nine. After working so passionately and hard to build my own small fitness business, I couldn't imagine a better situation; everything from the timing to the deal itself was perfect.

Two weeks passed and I saw no proposal. I followed up and received no response. I followed up again and again—and nothing. No response. The company's employees would come to my class and mention overhearing something about an expansion but still, no communication from the big guys. I felt unsteady. When was this going to happen? I mean, what about my future? When and how was I supposed to plan my life? I had been so excited and my dream had seemed so close; this was it! I would have signed a contract blindfolded!

I could have chosen to see the company's lack of response in terms of the dictionary definition of *problem* and regarded the entire situation as "harmful, something that needed to be overcome." By allowing their unresponsiveness to become a problem, I could have fallen into the trap of believing that their offer was the only way to achieve my goals. Seeing the partnership as the only shoe that fit could have left me anxious, frustrated, and stuck as I focused my energy entirely on attempting to "fix" things and make contact with the company.

Instead, I chose to see the situation through the eyes of my dad. In his mind, what some call a problem is actually a solution that isn't working. When it seems that something isn't working out the way you planned or hoped, it can be easy to forget what your original goals and intentions were. As my dad taught me, the turning point happens when you remember what you set out to do in the beginning and actually realize that your current problem used to be a solution. My original goal was to fill my time and add new meaning to my life; now I could see that selling my business to a larger company had been one way to accomplish that goal—but just one! There are *always* more ways to reach the goal.

My dad's concept of endless solutions allowed me to see a larger, more opportunity-filled world. With the ability to see the full range of possibility, I have now been able to approach another company about buying my fitness business, and write this book. Being open and feeling confident that other equal, if not better, solutions exist gives me the ability to recognize the vibrant, dynamic reality around me.

Over the years, I have found this lesson of my dad's invaluable. The solution to approach the fitness company was available before their unresponsiveness became a problem. The option of writing a book as a means to fill my time and add new meaning to my life was also available before the problem. Whether I choose to look back to the origin of my problems and see that they were once solutions or appreciate that untapped solutions are everywhere, the solution invariably exists *before* the problem.

You can also see that the "solution is born before the problem" because we seek out solutions for potential future "problems" all the time. From buying insurance on a new phone to carrying an umbrella for a rainy day, to accepting the death of a loved one, we are constantly thinking of potential solutions for our lives and ourselves. But, when we forget that the "solution was born before the problem," we get consumed by the problem and fail to discover and revel in a world filled with infinite solutions.

Truly embracing this lesson has given me a lively openness and an active acceptance that has changed my concept of problems and, as a result, my life. Like everyone, I still feel the emotions involved with problems but I now have the tools to quickly and resolutely bounce back, avoiding a prolonged attachment to the heaviness of those emotions. Because of my dad's lesson, my life feels consistently hopeful and my true self is calmer—I always know, no matter what the circumstance, that the solution existed before the problem. I just have to look.

"No one can take away your happiness."

Growing up, I saw disappointments in my father's life. Family took advantage of him, business partners stole from him, and he experienced death, betrayal, and countless other challenging situations. And yet he always said, "I'm happy."

Hearing this, I felt the same disbelief as when I was told there were no problems in the world, only solutions. I wondered what inspired him to say it. Was he lying? Was he in denial? Was he just trying to protect me? It was hard to understand because it made me question my own happiness. I didn't always feel happy— was there something wrong with me? Again, given time and experience, I understood this lesson. I not only deeply believe my father when he says he is happy, but I also constantly and genuinely say it myself.

Once, when I was nine years old, I was upset because I felt like I wasn't "cool" at school. I felt left out by the cool girls and thought that if I only figured out how to achieve coolness, I would be truly happy. I remember talking to my dad and he told me, "No one can take away your happiness."

Me: "I'm not happy because those girls don't think I'm cool."

Dad: "Honey, no one can take away your happiness."

Me: "What do you mean? They already have. Maybe they don't want me to be happy. Maybe they really don't like me. But I know I could be cool! I'm just not. I have to do something different."

Dad: "And, you think if you change who you are you'll be happy?"

Me: "Yes. I'll be more like them and we'll be friends. If I'm cool, I'll be happy and they'll be happy too!"

Dad: "Honey, you can't give away your happiness, either."

Me: "But, what if I want to and really mean it?"

Dad: "You still can't."

Me: "I do things to make you and Mommy happy, don't I?"

Dad: "No. We make ourselves happy."

I was only nine! His words seemed harsh. I remember feeling powerless, like I didn't have the influence I thought I did. I had already felt like I missed the sense of happiness everyone else seemed to have, and now I felt like my existence even at home was pointless. I was so confused by my father's response. I knew he loved me but he was telling me that who I was and what I did didn't change him. I had always thought there was a quick-fix solution to being happy and that I had a direct effect on others' happiness. But, for my father, happiness was a choice between the two following options:

Choosing to embrace the ability to control the way you experience life and ALLOWING yourself to feel emotions like pleasure or sadness from external factors.

OR

Choosing not to embrace your ability to control the way you experience life and REACTING with feelings like pleasure and sadness to external factors.

And, by using the word control, he wasn't indicating that I should force myself to feel something unnatural or unrealistic. Rather, he was encouraging me to surrender and accept my emotions in order to more effectively express and release them. *Allowing* myself to feel anger or sadness versus *reacting* with anger and sadness may seem like a subtle choice, but for my life, it's been the difference between happiness and unhappiness.

To better understand this lesson, consider the first lesson, "The solution is born before the problem." Since a solution always exists and finding it is an ability we can choose to embrace, we can also say that no one can take away our ability to find solutions. So, if the ultimate solution is happiness, then no one can take away our ability to find happiness. My happiness is <u>my</u> decision.

It comes down to this—we control our lives. My father chooses not to let external events and people affect his state of mind. Events and people *influence* him but he chooses how he will react to them. Essentially, he makes a choice to feel happy or unhappy. Although I am now grateful for my father's deeply ingrained theory that gave me the tools I needed to achieve happiness, when I was growing up, it was challenging.

For years, I felt anger and confusion when my dad would say, "No one can take away your happiness." In my own life, I experienced what seemed clearly to be unhappiness after fights with friends, bad grades, and kids picking on me. However, my parents seemed to be genuinely happy even after getting married without their parents' approval, coming to America with only $8, working five jobs between the two of them, and losing all of their hard-earned money in a fire that burned down their first business. Witnessing this resilience, their survivor mentality, and their unwillingness to surrender their own life and happiness to the outside world, I started to wonder.... Was it truly possible to have control over our own happiness? For me, it was only after a special trip to India to visit my grandmother that I began clearly to understand this lesson.

It was the summer of 1994 and I had not seen my grandmother in twelve years. The thought of traveling alone with my mom and visiting an old relative in an underdeveloped country wasn't exactly appealing. As a teenager, I was much more interested in staying at home with my friends and hanging out by the pool all day. But, I felt obligated to go. I received the required shots, bought new clothes, and took enough bug repellant to subdue an entire forest's insects. Although I was physically ready, nothing could have prepared me for the summer of surprises that unfolded.

My grandmother stood at a height of four feet, eight inches, a few inches shorter than me. She had beautiful long, gray hair, soft skin, and an irreplaceable and irresistible smile. Though she was small physically, her strong mentality was incredible; she could soar as high as the Himalayan Mountains! We created many memories that summer, staying up late talking and joking. Together, as grandmother and granddaughter, we lit up each other's hearts with electrifying love. We generously gave one another the love and attention we needed. I braided and oiled her hair every day, shaved her legs for the first time in her life, and she recited the Navkar Mantra, the most important Jain prayer that gives respect to all humans, with me every night. With admiration, I helped my grandma cook the traditional, tasteful sweets of India.

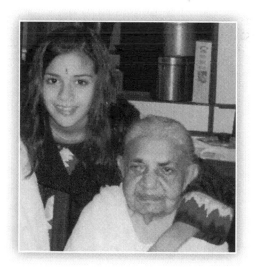

Although I loved my grandma's home-cooked meals, I still yearned for the quick fixes like candy, fruit, and chocolate from home. One day, I found a juicy, golden peach and quickly devoured it. It was sweet and satisfying; I found another one and ate it, too. Before our trip, my mom had warned me of the dangers of drinking the water in India; it didn't occur to me that the fruit that had been grown and washed there could also be potentially dangerous. But, these two peaches that seemed so trouble-free ended up pushing me to understand two difficult lessons from my parents.

After eating the peaches, I became the victim of a severe, deathly intestinal virus and, after a lengthy ordeal in India, I was forced to return to the U.S. a month earlier than planned. I was incredibly sad to have to cut short my precious time with my grandma. I cried as I said good-bye to her and I felt her tears come from a deep place in her heart; my grandmother knew she would not see my mother and me for years. I reflected on the inseparable bond we had created and vowed to return to India every year. She was my mother's mother, my sweet, special grandma, and she had a piece of my heart.

As soon as I got home, I made an audiotape for my grandma so she could hear the sound of my voice. I immediately mailed the tape to her in India. I knew she missed me as much as I missed her and that she would love the tape. Less than a month later, on August 28, 1994, she died in the same hospital bed I had suffered in, and by the same virus.

When I found out she died, I wanted to die. I felt guilty for not staying longer. I felt responsible for her death. I felt tormented.

Did she get the bug from me? Was I being taught a lesson? It was unsettling to think that I hadn't been there in twelve years and then the summer I decided to visit, she had died. I couldn't accept the fact that my widowed, aged grandmother, who had been reunited with youth in my presence, was gone. She was supposed to live until I could see her again; I was supposed to braid her hair again. Her loss bewildered my mind and darkened my soul.

I felt guilty for living. I locked myself in my bedroom for a week with the intention of staying there indefinitely. Since my grandmother had not been allowed to live, I felt I did not deserve to be happy in my own life. I refused to be happy in my daily routine because it seemed that the only respectable thing to do was stay still—essentially to stop living. Happiness didn't even seem to be an option anymore; it was as if my grandmother had taken it away with her when she died.

My father delicately guided me to understand that I could still be happy, because I was still in control—my grandmother couldn't take away my happiness and I couldn't give it to her. I was born with this control and I could choose to ignore or embrace it. I could still *feel* a full spectrum of emotions but I could choose how to let them influence my life. My dad encouraged me to take my time, to privately reflect, and to write a poem about my grandmother.

The choice was simple. I could choose to feel that I had no control and react uncontrollably and, as a result, feel perplexed, overwhelmed, suffocated, and consumed. Or I could choose to control my state of mind and allow myself to react the way I wanted to. I chose control—and as a result, I was able to make decisions about how I wanted to feel. I knew my grandmother wanted me to be happy, so I chose to allow myself to feel the overwhelming sadness of her death —but I also chose to feel compassion, strength, and acceptance. I took my dad's advice and with my newfound confidence, wrote a poem, which my dad encouraged me to submit to a national newspaper contest. I won the contest and received a certificate, and the poem was published in a book. I felt like my grandma would never be forgotten.

I found healing and a great resolve in this experience and in my dad's saying, "No one can take away your happiness." I am deeply grateful to my father for his patience and understanding during that time. It was his words and actions that inspired a priceless sense of freedom, strength, and validation in me.

My father always says, "Rupa, you are the captain of your soul and the driver of your own life." In my life, there WILL be obstacles, challenges and triumphs ahead—storms, sunny days, and the possibility of losing my way—but I know that I can always come back to my moral compass, check in, and steer my way towards happiness.

I see what I want to see on the road of life. I AM the driver. I have the power to stop, start, and refuel my car. I can stall. I can take shortcuts. I can choose each moment. It's so easy to put up walls and boundaries around our own freedom and build them so solidly that we feel as if they have always been there. We allow ourselves to get caught up in thinking we are stuck when in fact we *can* drive out. We can choose either to create our own road rage or the music we love to sing along to. My father's simple analogies and thoughtful advice have guided me in understanding the importance of choice and of embracing the ability I have to control the way I experience life.

I recently met a woman who made a documentary about happiness. She said the inspiration for the film came to her while she traveled through India. She was struck by the joy that seemed to emanate from the Indian people despite "all they lacked." When she told me this, I wondered about our different perceptions. Personally, I've been struck by just the opposite—people who can be happy despite "all they have," the external sources of happiness that Western society seems to rely so heavily upon.

Our lives are full of external sources of happiness such as material things, technology, and relationships with others. These sources are constantly evolving stimuli that seem to have the power to give or take away all of our happiness.

And, what is *happiness* anyway?

> **Happiness:** a state of contentment; a pleasurable or satisfying experience.

In my father's lesson, I've discovered an alternative definition for *happiness*.

> **Happiness:** a timeless state of contentment due to embracing the control you have over your state of mind.

From the point of view of this alternative perspective on happiness, it is hard to understand why the documentary filmmaker is so shocked by people who are happy with fewer external sources of happiness. Isn't it harder to be happy with so much stuff? Constantly being on the quest for more stuff can make your current physical or mental state feel inadequate. We've built our lives around acquiring new things and replacing things we've deemed as unsatisfying, and the transition from new to old is becoming quicker day by day. It's so tempting to go on the market for the newest, thinnest laptop soon after a recent purchase of a perfectly suitable one or casually hooking up at a party in search for love a day after a break-up. Whether it's a new computer or a new relationship, these external sources, although enjoyable, can distract us from our inner source of happiness. So, although my dad may be the number one fan of Apple, purchasing and using their products won't give him constant happiness. I was taught that finding happiness is two-fold—first, not getting distracted and attached to the unpredictable, tempting external sources, and second, not only knowing but embracing the only constant for hap-piness: the ability to control your state of mind, your internal source of happiness.

Seeing my own fluctuations over the years as well as others, I choose to embrace my ability to control my state of mind. My internal source of happiness is more reliable than any external source of happiness. I would rather be content no matter what—and also have the capacity to feel joy when I win a million dollars or feel deep sadness when someone close to me is gone.

So, the full lesson is this: no one can take away your happiness or give you happiness but YOU can take away happiness or give yourself happiness. That's a lot of power! Since you can choose to ignore it or embrace it, why not embrace it and begin living the happiest life possible?

"Don't magnify successes or failures."

My dad always has the last word. Whether it's on the phone or in person, there is always an old saying, a story from his childhood (the one you've heard a million times), or a repeated point. If I think the conversation is done, it's not. Being on the receiving end of constant feedback has felt comforting, challenging, and annoying. I can call my dad after feeling like I failed and am guaranteed a powerful vote of support and a realistic evaluation; the situation seems much more manageable after the phone call. I can also call my dad after feeling like I succeeded and be met with uninvited feedback and constructive criticism. His unsolicited support, advice, and persistent push to reflect make me feel the important impact of his lesson, "Don't magnify successes or failures."

This lesson is challenging because it requires me to find the delicate balance between my achievements and my disappointments. During times of failure, this lesson is incredibly comforting and during times of success, it is deeply humbling. No matter how much success or failure I experience in my life, my dad has a beautiful, unique way of making me see both my successes and failures as fleeting moments, nothing more and nothing less. With suggestions and insight he helps me realize that these moments are rich with lessons, exciting and rewarding, and that my perspective can transform my definition of them.

And if my outlook is the true determinant of success or failure, than I decide what is a "success" and what is a "failure."

Consider the definition of the word *magnify*.

> **Magnify:** make something larger than it is, especially with a lens or microscope.

To magnify something, to make it larger, is an intentional act that requires tools. Our tools—our body, mind and heart—are what we use to "see" the world. To magnify our successes or failures is to intentionally choose to make them bigger than they are—we use our mind and heart to do this. So, if we magnify our successes and failures, they end up being "bigger," more consuming moments, rather than just passing moments that fill up our lives.

Even though we are often taught to regard successes and failures as opposites, when we magnify them and attach ourselves to them, they can bring in equally destructive emotions. You could feel pressure to succeed or pressure for potential failure; you could feel entitled to a congratulations or entitled to sympathy; you could feel that you will never fail or feel that you will never succeed and be surprisingly unprepared for both. You could restrict yourself by magnifying your successes and failures or you could choose not to magnify them and feel freedom. And with that freedom comes the ability to accurately evaluate, actively appreciate, and genuinely accept all moments in life—the successes and the failures. My dad offered me the tools to see that success and failure are not only equal in what they can offer us, but, like other elements of life, are to be expected.

I have learned that his purpose in sharing this lesson is not to dim the light of success or ignore the sting of failure but rather to encourage an autonomy that exists when you are unattached to outcomes. He encourages me to be thankful for my journey towards a goal and appreciative of the best AND worst that could occur along the way.

My father strongly believes that if we choose to magnify, we get attached to the successes and failures of others and ourselves. We begin to see successes and failures as definitions of character and overall achievement. We disregard feelings of humility, forgiveness, love, sharing, and teaching—the requirements for growth that truly define our humanity. In fact, magnifying successes and failures stunts our growth and isolates us. If I magnify and define my life or others' lives by focusing on successes and failures, I will attach myself to increased feelings of entitlement, pressure, and insecurity. And as a result, I will hold myself back from fully sharing in and enjoying other people's lives and being truly happy with my own life.

It's easy to give examples of huge life moments as successes and failures: losing a job, getting the job of your dreams, breaking up, having a long-relationship; they are the kind that stand out. And my dad's first two lessons, "The solution is born before the problem" and "No one can take away your happiness," apply to these big moments in your life. When looking at these first two lessons with introspection, big moments no longer have to be defined as successes or failures. "Don't magnify successes or failures" actually comes down to the power of small moments and how we choose to define them. Two experiences from my childhood demonstrate this and show how this lesson can be applied to all moments, no matter how small

When I was in third grade, my teacher called my parents to tell them that I was not only disruptive but that math was extremely difficult for me. She was personally discouraged and not hopeful about my progress. My father could have chosen to magnify this and to see me as lacking something—but he didn't. He sat down with me and said that when he has trouble learning things, sometimes all he needs is a different approach. He helped me photocopy each page of my math book and said I could even make a new cover for the book and call it whatever I wanted. We went through the "new" book every night; my dad dedicated time to helping me learn new approaches to math. Without pressure or attachment, he reassured me that all he expected was for me to try, to tell him when I didn't understand something, and to trust him. I did, and after six months, math became my favorite subject. My dad didn't magnify this "failure"; he saw it as a moment, helped me in an encouraging, loving way, and we moved on.

Another third grade experience: I loved dancing and wanted to be a ballerina . Though I was usually very nervous about being on stage, at this particular end-of-year performance at my ballet school, I shone! I received many compliments and was so proud of myself. I asked my dad repeatedly if I was the best. He told me he was proud of me and wanted to know each detail of my experience and how I felt. He forced me to focus on the experience rather than the outcome. The next day, my family and I watched my dad's video of the performance; I could see on his face how proud he was of me but also how happy he was for other kids and their families. He had videotaped not only me but every other performer as well.

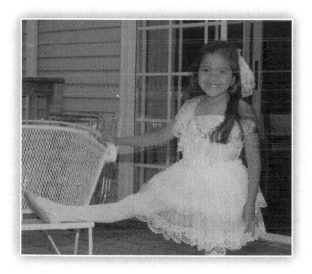

We all watched as every dancer did their best; everyone was the best. He chose not to magnify my "success" and as a result, I felt closer to the other girls who had also succeeded. I appreciate my dad's admirable capacity for love. When you can see that the world is full of not only your own successes and failures, but others' as well, you feel more comforted. Not only can you relate to people you know but you can connect to strangers as well, because we ALL experience success and failure.

Without this lesson, small successes and failures can turn into larger issues, bringing in unbalanced egos, uncompromising viewpoints, and misinterpreted securities. My dad believes that this saying, "Don't magnify successes and failures," greatly contributes to his healthy, 46-year marriage to my mom. My dad and mom can come home and say to each other, "I messed up" and know that they have each other's support and that the moment will pass. They also know that if they come home with successes they will be met with excitement, solicited (as well as unsolicited) insight, and loving space to potentially fail. This non-attachment and freedom helps maintain a delicate balance of happiness in my home.

Unlike my dad's sayings, which as a child I often found shocking and tough to understand, my mom's self-created mantras seemed simple to digest. I've realized that this is far from the truth. My dad's lessons, although difficult to initially comprehend, after time and reflection, now feel instinctual. Conversely, my mom's lessons seemed easy initially but now, after time and reflection, seem more difficult. I continue to see the ever-growing complexity and deep meaning in each one.

My dad's drive towards happiness inspires him to persevere and define life on his own terms. My mom, on the other hand, is driven by balance and you'll see that her one word allows her to understand and accept life on her own terms. She is strong and has resolute faith in spirituality. It is this non-negotiable spiritual strength that makes her mantras the key to her life's balance. Her lessons require self-control, faith in humanity, and patience.

My mom's lessons are like opening a pomegranate, rich with flavor but time-consuming, challenging and have many layers. Understanding them requires acceptance; you must be prepared to dig deep to understand them completely. I truly believe you will find worth; her careful use of simple words unexpectedly invites you to find an intricate and powerful meaning.

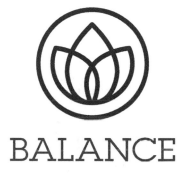

BALANCE

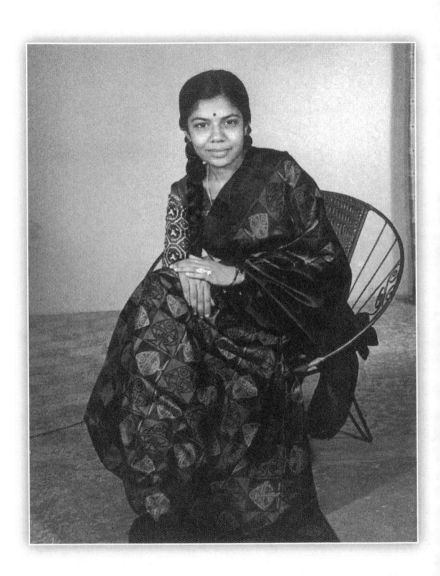

Mom

I love listening to my mom speak. She has an endearing, youthful cheer in her voice that's coupled perfectly with the comforting tone of a wise, old soul. She makes herself laugh and laughs often. This light-heartedness, balanced with her deep wisdom, makes you want her by your side during ordinary conversations and in hard times as well. If my mom were an object, she would be the comforting, faithful, warm "blankie" I slept with as a child. And just as I grew out of needing my blankie, in time, after my mom's comfort, I was expected to grow up.

She promotes independence. So many times in my life, after much motherly comfort, suddenly, my blankie will be gone and I'll be standing on my own two feet. My mom will hand me her umbrella before the first storm, stand strongly by my side when the storm hits, and help me appreciate the calm afterward. However, when the second storm comes, she'll expect and push me to stand on my own. At every moment in my life, my mom has both nurtured and encouraged me to find my independence. My mom, Nalini Pinak Mehta, epitomizes balance.

My mom was born and raised in Ahmadabad, India. She grew up in a wealthy and deeply religious home and was raised to be a mild-mannered, traditional Indian woman.

My grandmother's traditional and devout religious ambitions and my grandfather's challenging and modern ways created a balanced upbringing that greatly influenced my mom's character and journey.

Religion was the first priority for my Jain grandmother; she would wake up at five a.m. every day to pray, and her goal was to create a strict, devotional home. Although small, Jainism, an ancient Dharmic religion, has a strong influence in India and prescribes a path of non-violence toward all forms of living beings in the world. From eggs to carrots, true Jain followers do not eat any animal products or any food grown beneath the ground. My grandmother took pride in being Jain and was my mother's role model of tradition and faith.

My grandfather was a successful businessman, highly respected in his community. After growing up poor and creating his own success, he had a dignified presence, exemplified by his pressed suits, chauffeurs, and the signa-ture green ink he used to write his telegrams. Though uneducated, he was progressive for 1930s India. He took his daughters on trips to see the country and enrolled them in the best boarding school. For five years, my mom attended school where she prayed, practiced yoga and meditation daily, and washed her own clothes. She received visits from her parents monthly. My mom still talks about this time as the best time of her life and still proudly remembers graduating at the top of her class. At home or school, my mom took pride in being a model student and an obedient child. My mom's hero was my grandfather because of his success, poise, and contemporary outlook.

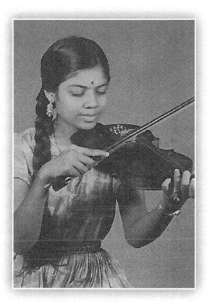

Growing up, my mom had aspirations of becoming a doctor. But because such a commitment would affect her getting married at an "appropriate" age, her mother encouraged her to go to art school instead. Despite the glimpse of independence offered by my grandfather, my mom was raised to be a traditional Indian woman, one who would study art, not science, have an arranged marriage, and eventually live with her husband's parents. However, nothing could have prepared her family for this future event: marrying a poor jungle boy from a different caste and religion out of love rather than arrangement.

How did a wealthy, studious, and obedient Jain girl even cross paths with a poor, adventurous Hindu boy? A bus.

My mom was 22 when she boarded the bus for home like any other day. My father, who happened to be on the bus, already knew who she was; his younger brother, who was dating my mom's younger sister, had pointed her out to him. (My mom didn't even know her sister was dating, yet eventually these two brothers would marry the sisters!) My mom sat down on the bus and was prepared to pay the conductor, but when he came over, he said her ticket was already paid for—a gentleman in the back of the bus had bought it. In her timid, compliant style, she did not even turn around to see who the man was and kept reading her book! That evening she told her sister about the mystery man on the bus. Her sister already knew what had happened and arranged for them to formally meet.

My mom started seeing my dad, sneaking to movies, going for walks with him, and liked him, but their courtship was difficult; my grandfather introduced her and my aunt to potential suitors almost daily, and she was ridden with guilt. She was supposed to be a "good" woman but now she was not only dating a boy behind her father's back, but he was a poor boy from a different caste and religion. She wanted to please her father but she was in love with my dad. She was the most respectful and academic daughter and now she was doing something that seemed unforgivable.

At this time in India, an arranged marriage was the only option; a love marriage without family involvement was unheard of. Feeling unable to face her father, she fearfully wrote him a letter. She wrote of her love for my dad and how she couldn't marry any of the other men she had been introduced to. After receiving the letter, my grandfather invited my father to his office and told him to treat my mom like his sister, not his future wife. My dad respectfully said he couldn't do that. My grandfather then put restrictions in place, from locking windows and doors to preparing to send my mom and aunt to a rural town to marry and settle down. The pressure, timing, and her little sister's relationship with my dad's younger brother pushed my obedient mom to unpredictably run away from home with her sister.

Police and family frantically looked for the two sisters. There was drama, tears, anger, judgment, and sadness. With the coaxing of my mom's older sisters and their husbands, who my grandfather deeply respected, my grandparents eventually accepted my father. To this day, my mom still cries when she thinks of the worry and pain she caused her hero, her father.

From the bus ride that started it all, to their complicated and emotional marriage, only six months had passed, but finally my parents settled into a routine in Mumbai. My dad had a successful job; my brother was born and they were building their life as a family. But before long, my seemingly delicate mom felt the need for another great change in her life.

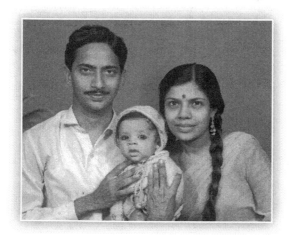

My mom had always been drawn to America, the land of opportunity where she believed her family could have the liberties she herself had been unable to have in traditional India. My mom made a decision to move. Although my dad had a great job and they were near both of their families, because of her undeniably potent inner voice, my mom knew she had to come to America, just like she knew she had to marry my dad. My mom's moral compass strengthened her and over the years continues to guide her to an inner peace that she ultimately trusts. So with her resolve, she chose to wait patiently and to faithfully convince my dad for years to try for a visa to come to America. He eventually did, and now, my Indian mom can say she has been a proud American for forty-one years.

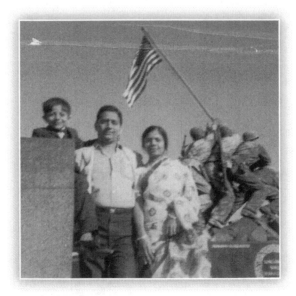

My mom is a perfect balance of East and West. She is traditional and modern, open-minded and opinionated, selfish and selfless, timid and courageous, humble and confident, religious and worldly. She is Indian. She is American. She uniquely embodies Indian confidence, vision, adaptability, and faith and embraces American independence, lifestyle, and opportunities.

My mom quickly adapted to American life. She found the few Indian grocery stores and stocked her kitchen, changed her name to Nikki (Nalini was hard for many to say), and applied for jobs. Although this life was so far from what her father had planned for her, the vision of freedom and opportunity for her family drove her. It motivated her to overcome every obstacle; washing my dad's only dress shirt daily for work, learning English, and increasing her math skills to become a bank teller, real estate agent, retail manager, and eventually an accountant. And still, she managed to cook traditional Indian food (bread from scratch!) for her husband and children every day. I remember my mom, despite working full-time, cooking a big breakfast and full course dinner daily until I moved to college. And in spite of some adolescent jumpiness, each meal was at the dining table where her children had to talk about their day and current events with the family.

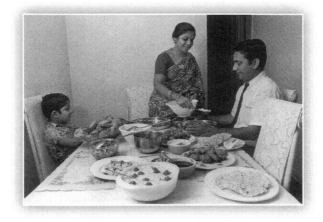

She even learned to cook meat and made excellent beef dishes for us so we would feel comfortable eating American cheeseburgers with friends. I was completely shocked to find out five years ago that she had actually grown up in a strict vegan home. It was only after I moved out and went to college that she returned to her vegan upbringing.

Just as my mom adapted to American food, she also embraced and celebrated American holidays and traditions. I have celebrated Thanksgiving, Christmas, Easter, and Hanukkah in addition to Indian holidays since I was a child. From decorating our home with 10,000 lights in December to painting eggs in April, any time there was a reason to celebrate and learn, my parents were there, sharing and enjoying the experience to the fullest.

Growing up with the ideal of having an arranged marriage and becoming a mother and housewife who nurtures her family through religion, food, and sacrifice, I find it incredible that my mom has achieved a balance in challenging her upbringing while maintaining it admirably. My mom has a strict vegetarian diet, prays every morning and night, wears traditional Indian clothing, cooks homemade Indian breads, soups, and vegetables daily, speaks in her native tongue to her family, watches Zee TV (the Indian channel), maintains relationships with her family in India, and exceptionally upholds Indian holidays and traditions. But she is also a successful accountant, manages several small businesses, handles the family's finances, doesn't pressure me to get married, encourages me as an entrepreneur, supports my traveling alone, and welcomes anyone of any caste or background into our home.

Upon meeting my mom, you would be touched by her motherly love and genuine sweetness, and humbled by her drive and wisdom. My mom drums to her own beat and loves and trusts herself greatly. As a result, she loves her life, is confident in her decisions, and faithfully believes in the way she raised her children. In my eyes, my mom has the character of Mother Teresa, the values of Mahatma Gandhi (her second hero), and the innocence of a child.

My mom's soft strength is reflected in her voice, her actions, and even her food.

Her all-American Aunt Jemima pancakes with a kick of zucchini, green pepper, and Indian mango chutney is one of my favorite dishes. And, if my mom could, she would share this dish, among many others deliciously made with love, with everyone in her home. If you were a guest at our dinner table, you would enjoy an abundance of homemade food, hear my mom's laughter and feel the warmth of her nurturing welcome.

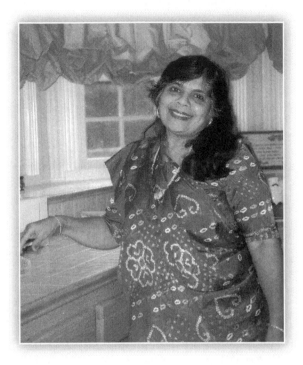

"Shut up. Sit. Smile."

For me, "Shut up. Sit. Smile." is the hardest lesson from my mom. If you knew me, you would know that the phrase "shut up" doesn't sound like something I would say or do, "sitting" is something I rarely do, and "smiling" is something I do easily but never consciously.

As I mentioned in a previous lesson, the two peaches I ate in India resulted in a deadly intestinal virus. There I was, in India, becoming so close to my grandmother, eating fruit one day and being hospitalized the next day. For me, this difficult sequence of events helped me gain insight into two important lessons from my parents, my dad's lesson "No one can take away your happiness" and this, my mom's lesson, "Shut up. Sit. Smile." Her lesson was and still is challenging. However, the episode of the memorable Indian peaches, one of the most challenging experiences of my life, led me to understand it better.

Eating the peaches caused me to vomit uncontrollably and lose twenty pounds and the ability to walk. I hadn't spent much time in hospitals and had never been in one filled with insects, lizards, and no running water. The doctors gave us mixed messages—I could get better with treatment, time, and rest or I could get worse. The doctors were confused by my symptoms. I spent long nights lying on cold hospital beds and warmed myself with con-versations with the kind nurses. My mom stayed all day and night with me and I could see that she was scared I was going to die.

The idea of death became as common as getting up and brushing my teeth. I really thought that this was it—my life was going to be over in sixteen short years, wrapped up with daily intravenous tubes, bottles, and hourly shots. My mom and I saw patients die before our eyes and heard the helpless cries and worries. Everyday, it shook me more and more. My need for human contact and for life increased. The conditions in the hospital felt worse than death. I had come to India to sightsee and what I was experiencing instead was terrifying. I didn't want this; I just wanted to see the Taj Majhal!

My vacation became the time I spent with the warm nurses and my sweet grandmother—they were my escape from the struggle. As we became closer, they began to represent heal-ing and spirituality for me. My feelings for them grew into an indestructible emotional strength that helped combat my fears. The unforgettable days I spent with these loving people and the bonds that developed were more fulfilling and powerful than any monument or temple I could have seen.

After suffering four erratic and scary weeks in the hospital, the doctors gave me clearance and orders to immediately board a plane to the US. After I was released from the hospital, we returned to my uncle's house and prepared for the voyage back to America. I showered, put fresh clothes on, and was ready to go back to the hospital to say goodbye to the special people I had met. I was so excited for them to see my clean face and give them my American CDs and other gifts. I wanted to show them how much I appreciated and would miss them. I happily hopped into the car with my mom, but I was met with an unwelcome surprise.

My mom said we were not going to say goodbye! We were not going to the hospital; instead we were going straight to the airport. Given the hospital's conditions and my fragile state, she thought I would get sick again if I went back. I thought she was being selfish and ungrateful; I tried to hurt her by saying rude things. And, that day, I said the meanest things I've ever said to my mom before deciding to not speak to her until we were home, a total of three days. Later I saw that while my intention was to be appreciative of the people who had helped me, it was unfair to my mom; she was saying goodbye to her family and preparing for a long flight from India to America with an angry child who had just barely survived four weeks in the hospital.

Despite my mean words, my attempts to cause guilt, and my obnoxiously "loud" three-day "silence", the only thing my patient mom said was, "Rupa, I love you. This is for your best interest and your anger will eventually pass. Remember, if you shut up and sit, the smile will come." I was infuriated. I was shutting up, hoping to prove a point to my mom—and instead it was proving her point! I was sitting because I had to and I definitely couldn't see any of this resulting in a smile. I was so angry with her, how would this pass?

These actions, *shut up*, *sit,* and *smile*, felt so forced. They felt like duct tape across my mouth and spirit, aggressively holding me down and forcing me to sit when I had so much to say. And a smile was in the realm of impossible.

Before I embraced this lesson, the words, *shut up, sit* and *smile* seemed to have such easy definitions; my comprehension of them was second nature. However, when I looked deeper into these "obvious" definitions through the balanced eyes of my mom, I found a powerful tool for love and a priceless lesson in self-control and empathy.

First, the ordinary definitions.

> **Shut up:** informal stop; cause someone to stop talking.

> **Sit:** adopt or be in a position in which one's weight is supported by one's buttocks rather than one's feet.

> **Smile:** a pleased, kind, or amused facial expression, typically with the corners of the mouth turned up and the front teeth exposed.

Now, consider my mom's altered definitions.

> **Shut up:** turn off your mind chatter, your repetitive, debilitating thoughts; cultivates self-control.

Sit: relax and release; cultivates being grounded.

Smile: make something more pleasant, "lighter"; cultivates the ability to listen.

Oh...

My mom's lesson was not, "Rupa, stop talking, sit there festering, and force yourself to smile."

Her lesson was much deeper and more difficult than that. "Shut up. Sit. Smile." meant, "Rupa, find your self-control and turn off your mind chatter; sit and be present; listen, and eventually things will become lighter."

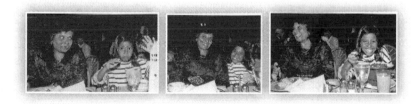

So, why did she offer the lesson in such blunt, simplistic terms? Why didn't she just say, "Be present and listen"? Because regardless of the difference between the dictionary definitions and my mom's, she knew that it would feel forced and I would immediately reject it. She knew it would take practice and hard-hitting words for me to realize the potential of this lesson. My mind was frantic, my passion high, and my ability to hide my feelings non-existent. I <u>needed</u> to "Shut up. Sit. Smile."

We have all been in emotionally charged situations with people we care about. Whether the dialogue is spoken or passive or the blame is placed on you or them, the situation can benefit from my mom's simple mantra, "Shut up. Sit. Smile."

I was in a relationship in which there was a lot of tension and hurt between my boyfriend and me. Even though we talked about it, very little got resolved. When I wasn't satisfied with our interactions, felt there was nothing I could do that I hadn't tried already, and felt like saying things that I would later regret, I remembered this lesson from my mom—and it worked! Forcing myself to "Shut up. Sit. Smile." allowed the tough moments to freely pass from tension to understanding. If I don't get in the way of stressed situations with my own reaction and really find the empathy to listen, the situation will calm down and move forward, just as it did with my mom.

My mom's lesson has shown me that the capacity to move forward has to do with quieting the noise in your mind, truly being in the moment, and listening. Sometimes it is difficult; sometimes you have to force yourself to shut up and sit there, even though you're aching to move and speak. You have to force yourself to be open even though you feel closed. But this can be the quickest way to quieting the storm and attaining a sense of internal calm. If you can find the self-control and empathy to stay in the moment, the heavy situation will begin to lighten, become clear, and a smile from within will start to surface naturally. Eventually, you'll rip off the "duct tape" and find a genuine smile underneath!

"Love yourself dearly. Be yourself completely. Treat yourself occasionally."

I recently ended a loving three-year relationship with a wonderful man. We had tried everything—communication, therapy, vacation, time apart—anything that we thought could bring down the unhealthy level of intensity upon which the relationship was founded. But nothing worked. We went through a gut-wrenching, tough, amicable, and respectful breakup. We sadly told our families who had become incredibly close and I moved out of the homey apartment we had excitedly bought and successfully renovated together three years before. I came to this pivotal decision after a long and emotional internal struggle—I had loved this man immensely and dreamed of having a future with him but my true spirit did not want to be in the relationship.

About six months before the relationship ended, my mom and I had an important conversation. My boyfriend and I were spending the weekend with my family and everybody seemed to be enjoying the time together. But, he and I had been fighting more and more and I found myself hiding behind closed doors the entire weekend, stressfully thinking about my future.

My mom, with a calm reserve, spoke to me in the kitchen one morning. She said, "Rupa, if you get married one day and you are struggling and feel in your heart it isn't working, don't worry too much. And, if I'm not around but you feel you need my approval or support to end it or get a divorce, you don't. We're in America now—you can do anything. I trust the way I raised you. You have the tools to love yourself and be happy. And, I will always love you but I'll always give you advice while I'm here. I mean I AM your mom. I love your boyfriend but I love you more and if you want advice on how to make it work or not work let me know. Remember: Love yourself dearly. Be yourself completely. Treat yourself occasionally."

I had heard this mantra before from my mom but when she said it that day, she generously showed me that I could offer myself simplicity, insightfulness, and compassion. I was at a point where I wanted to start the brave and liberating task of ending the relationship but I didn't know where to begin. When my mom saw me that weekend, she instinctively knew that I needed less self-questioning and more, loving guidance.

Whenever I am going through a difficult time, I find great comfort in this mantra. I feel like I'm in my mom's kitchen watching her lovingly put butter into everything and I feel her warmth. I repeat her words to myself and just saying them, I know that I'm taking the first step towards resolving my dilemma and healing myself after a trying time. For me, the comfort in this lesson, "Love yourself dearly. Be yourself completely. Treat yourself occasionally.," is in the adverbs. Her intentional choice of the words *dearly, completely,* and *occasionally* truly ignites this powerful lesson in balance.

Let's take a look at the dictionary definitions of the first two, *dearly* and *completely*.

> **Dearly:**   with much affection, at a great cost.

> **Completely:**   totally, utterly.

My mom makes it clear that *dearly* and *completely* have different meanings and serve different purposes. The mantra is not "Love and be yourself completely." It is, "Love yourself *dearly*. Be yourself *completely*." Loving myself completely, totally, and utterly is not the goal. For my mom, *dearly* implies a fulfilling love that is whole-hearted but comes at an essential cost: embracing and owning up to my role in my life, including my flaws and mistakes. This means taking responsibility for my actions, apologizing when necessary, and saying thank you without an ego. When I own up to my life, I can allow my true self to be revealed entirely without hiding, blaming, being defensive, or feeling insecure. It's only when I love myself *dearly* that I can be myself *completely*.

When I finally did decide to end the relationship, I kept asking myself if I had failed in some way. I felt guilty, angry, and wondered if I would ever meet someone else or if anyone could ever love me again. My mom did not discourage me from asking questions, but she encouraged me to think of her mantra, "Love yourself dearly. Be yourself completely. Treat yourself occasionally." as a unifying theme I could come back to. I would eventually have to face my partner's actions as well as my own in the relationship, find my own voice, and move on. My questions were leading me to feel disconnected from my contribution, the situation, and myself. But after my mom helped me to love myself *dearly* and be myself *completely*, I was able to quiet the noise in my mind and truly connect again; I was able to move back to my core.

My mom was trying to balance my questions with answers. She wanted me to see that I could question myself repeatedly with self-doubt but I could also answer my own questions. In fact, I could answer each one, move on, and give myself freedom, love, and balance. Introspection and awareness were valuable, but dwelling on certain feelings and decisions that had been made was not loving or encouraging.

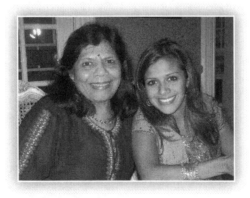

I needed to ask myself if there was something both of us could have done better but also remember what both of us had done well. My mom strongly feels that feeling guilty and angry keeps you stuck in the past. If you make a mistake, take responsibility, apologize, and move on with the pledge to do better in the future. And, wondering if anyone could ever love me again, I was reminded of my dad's lesson, "No one can take away your happiness." If I have the power to take away and give myself happiness, then I must also have the power to take away and give myself love. My relationships, decisions, emotions, and actions are all reflective of me and ultimately, I have the tools to love myself *dearly* and be myself *completely*.

Although the essence of being yourself *completely* is healthy and empowering, my mom believes it can be deceiving as well, overshadowing the rest of the lesson. The lesson is only complete when all three aspects are embraced equally, the last being, "Treat yourself occasionally."

Let's look at the dictionary definition of *occasionally*.

Occasionally: occurring, appearing, or done infrequently and irregularly; produced on or intended for a special occasion.

Again, my mom makes a clear distinction between *occasionally* and *completely*. The mantra isn't "Be and treat yourself completely." It is "Be yourself *completely*. Treat yourself *occasionally*." Her concern is that I could get caught up in thinking that if I am myself completely, I am allowed to treat myself completely. So, what's wrong with that? Well, if I only think of myself and forget about my surroundings, people, and ultimate goals, I might be foolish and indulgent. I could treat myself all the time (completely) and justify it with "I deserve it, I earned it, and I want it." So, she taught me to treat myself *occasionally,* not *completely.*

For me, "Treat yourself occasionally" is the icing on top of this lesson. My mom always says, "Rupa, when your spirit is in need of a hug, it's nice to treat yourself. So, go get some ice cream, a new pair of sneakers, or hang with your friends and play games. Go enjoy something full of pleasure. But, Rupa, don't do it too much." My mom wants me to understand that I can pick myself up for a moment or two with external things, but doing so isn't the long-lasting path to being myself. Ultimately, being myself isn't using external sources of happiness to define myself—going to a yoga class, buying the new iphone, or blocking out an entire relationship. If I focus too much on these external things, I lose the internal; I lose the person I am on the inside. I am myself *completely* only when I am not sidetracked by the external and am able to turn my focus inward and find my true spirit.

When we tap into our inner spirit, we embrace and accept the parts we like and don't like, building our self-confidence. The benefits are long-lasting and profound when we acknowledge but don't focus on our external sources of happiness and instead focus on our internal sources of happiness. During my break-up, I thought I was looking deep into my spirit with my questions, but I was actually distracting myself from my spirit with strong, relentless mind chatter. Truly looking inward and having the tools from my mom to intently listen to my spirit rather than getting caught up in the external noise is something I cherish. "Love yourself dearly. Be yourself completely. Treat yourself occasion- ally." means letting my spirit shine through with no judgment or self-abuse but with balanced reflection and self-control.

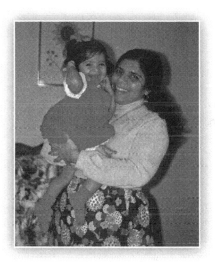

In one of the most difficult times of my life, my mom empowered me with this mantra. And now I offer this mantra, "Love yourself dearly. Be yourself completely. Treat yourself occasionally.," my blankie to you; sometimes life is hard and scary and you just want a blankie. Say this mantra to yourself; it will offer you comfort and help you on the path to standing on your own two feet again.

"Let go. Love. Live."

After several years in corporate America, my only sibling, my brother, chose to work for my father in his heating and air conditioning business. My analytical, practical, smart, and experienced brother teamed up with my dad's small business. This was my dad's dream—his only son, who he respected and loved greatly, choosing the family business over a corporate job! Filled with big ideas and much excitement about this father–son venture, my father couldn't have been happier.

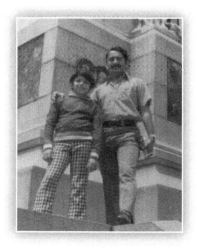

It started out well, but like many other family businesses, the working relationship was complicated and quickly became negative. As work issues came home to both houses, repressed emotions came out. My mom felt that the stresses between father and son could become dangerous to their close relationship and, in the best interest of the family, she fired my brother while offering to support him financially for as long as he needed. My brother, experiencing a range of understandable emotions, refused to talk to my parents for three years. Three years!

This family experience still astonishes me. I lived with my parents during most of this time and never once heard or felt a sense of regret, anger, judgment, or lack of faith that my brother would speak to them again. How did they let go like that? Didn't they feel like they didn't deserve that? How did they go from talking to my brother every single day to not at all? Didn't they feel like proving a point or encouraging guilt in my brother for his actions? They didn't.

My mom had faith in my brother and in herself. Because she "loved herself dearly" and "was herself completely," she was able to attentively and genuinely listen to my brother. My mom followed her mantras of "Love yourself dearly. Be yourself completely. Treat yourself occasionally." and "Shut up. Sit. Smile." and was able to truly let go. For her, truly letting go means accepting people, situations, and realities rather than holding on to them. Sometimes we falsely let go, thinking we've moved on when, in actuality, we're still trying to maintain control. My mom might have learned to *deal* with my brother's distance but the intensity and heaviness of the situation would have been rehashed over and over again. She wouldn't have truly accepted his choice and it could have been detrimental to their relationship.

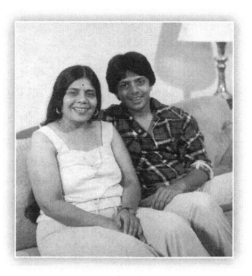

I was taught that when letting go seems impossible, it could be beneficial to think of the consequences of holding on. Therefore, let's look at the definitions of the antonyms of *let go, love* and *live - hold on, hate,* and *dead—.*

> **Hold on:** endure or continue in difficult circumstances.

> **Hate:** feel intense or passionate dislike; have a strong aversion to.

> **Dead:**   no longer alive; having lost sensation.

Holding on, as opposed to letting go, causes a lack of movement, intense feelings (often of dislike or even hate), and manifests into a life lacking energy and vitality (dead). Holding on impacts the happiness of your life. If I want to live a happy life and unlock the tight grip I could have on all of life's numerous little and big things—a friend not calling back, a mean comment, a person taking my seat on the train, loved ones not under-standing me—then I have to let go.

I offer this lesson from my mom last because her previous lessons, "Shut up. Sit. Smile." and "Love yourself dearly. Be yourself completely. Treat yourself occasionally." are requirements to learning this last, interdependent, enlightened lesson in trust and faith. And my mom's three lessons are what have led to my parents and brother having one of the most special and honest relationships I have ever witnessed.

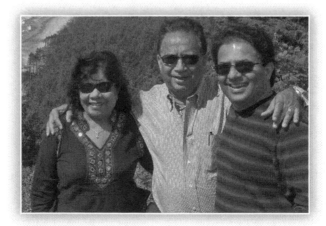

Life happens. You'll make mistakes; others will make mistakes. You'll ask for forgiveness; others will ask you for forgiveness. You'll want to be loved; others will want you to love them. You'll want people to listen; others will want you to listen. Stuff happens and more stuff will happen. Life has a cycle.

"Let go. Love. Live." is a cyclical lesson.

To *let go*, you must *live* and *love*.
To *love*, you must *let go* and *live*.
To *live*, you must *let go* and *love*.

And the cycle will continue.

So, the choice is to either *hold on*, *hate* and *die* or *let go*, *love* and *live*. When you hold on with a stagnant state of mind, you don't have the healthy momentum to move forward, let go, love, and live a fulfilling life. And even though I've been hurt, made mistakes, felt misunderstood, and have the ability to fight back, I choose to let go. I choose to love and live.

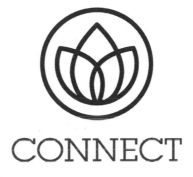

CONNECT

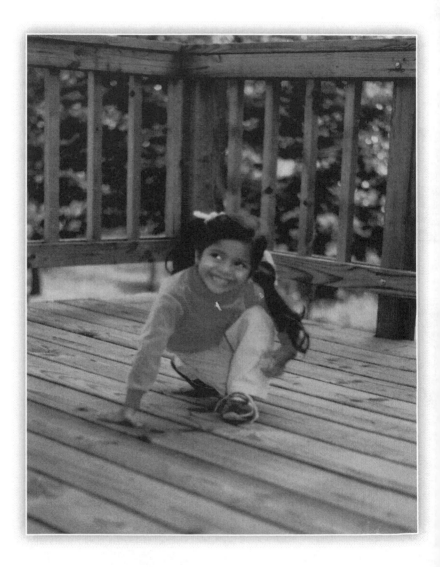

"Say thank you."

Our culture loves to say thank you. From Hallmark cards to 1-800-flowers, we have companies built on the premise that favorable thoughts and expressions of gratitude are good. We say thanks to the waitress, the lunch lady, the teacher, the President, and God. But, why don't we say thank you to the parents who gave us a foundation to build our lives upon?

To be fair, we do thank our parents lovingly around birthdays, anniversaries, and holidays. But the term "thank you" seems different somehow when we truly contemplate our upbringing. Take a look at the definition of *thank*.

> **Thank:** 1) express gratitude to (someone).
>
> 2) used ironically to assign blame or respon-sibility for something.

For me, reading part two of the definition was astonishing, but in the context of our culture, it does begin to make sense. When it comes to American culture, parents, and upbringings, we tend to assign blame or responsibility to our parents for our life's failures. And what about our successes? Oh... we take full credit for those.

My parents always say, "The only thing constant in life is change and death." Growing up with this as a foundation was difficult. Talking so freely about the unreliability of things and people I loved and the inevitability of death led to conversations that often seemed cold, hopeless, and even taboo. But now, if I keep the meaning behind this quote in my heart, I can truly understand the cycle of life and death and the importance of thanking my parents. They are people I love and one day they will be gone; I want to recognize this cycle and appreciate them for what they have given me.

I thanked my parents all the time as a little girl, looking at them with big, admiring eyes; I didn't thank them in high school as a rebellious teenager; I did thank them when they supported me in college; I didn't thank them when they didn't fully agree with my career choices; I do thank them now. Thanking and appreciating people, especially our parents, comes in cycles. The emotions and realities I associate with my parents are not constants; they will change in conjunction with where I am in my life. To understand this is to embrace the saying, "The only thing constant in life is change and death."

And, this is why "Say thank you" is *my* lesson. Our parents were once children like us. And we may someday be (or may already be) parents ourselves. It is a choice to either ignore or accept this beautiful cycle. Our parents will die and so will we. So, accept the cycle, embrace your motivation when it happens, and because words do matter, make an active effort to say thanks to your parents,

I don't always understand my parents nor do I agree with their every word and action; that would be impossible and is not the natural cycle of life. But no matter what, my parents' challenging lessons are part of my journey, my cycle, and my life. I can choose to define them the way I want to and now, I choose to feel truly lucky and thankful. And, because their words have shaped my life, I say the words "thank you" to them.

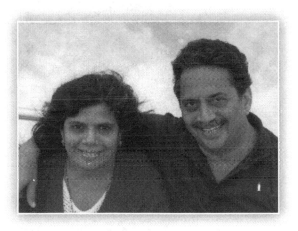

Accepting this cycle has caused me to expect the unexpected. Because I expect that my feelings and attitudes towards my upbringing and my parents will consistently change over time, I feel lighter on my path to understanding my past and letting go of unanswered questions and inert emotions. Things from my life journey don't have to feel "heavy" and unchangeable; things can, will, and do pass.

Losing the emotional weight of childhood and understanding the weight of words, allows me to connect to my true self. And although I aspire to embrace my mom's gift of balance and my dad's gift of happiness; I've accepted my own gift. Thankfully, my parents taught me to be *happy* with my own gift and I want to *balance* my lucky life by sharing that gift with others. My dad's life in one word, *happiness*, and my mom's life in one word, *balance*, have led me to the one word that defines and drives my life—*connect*.

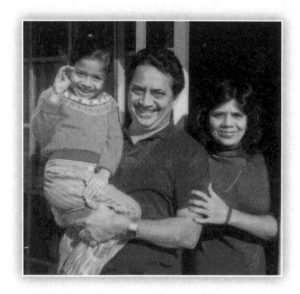

Ever since I was a little girl, I have wanted to connect. Whether it was joining numerous arts classes and participating in sports with other kids, sharing my toys, constantly inviting people to my house, or talking non-stop to anyone that would listen, I have always thrived on connecting to people, even imaginary people! As a child, I pretended to have more siblings just to play a more connected form of make believe. But beyond people, I continue to ask myself questions about my connection to the world. Why am I the way I am? Why did I choose to live in New York? How do other people grow up? Why did I become a teacher? What are the life experiences of others? Why did I write this book? My drive to connect with people and to my life experiences is what makes the word—connect— resonate within me.

When I'm unmotivated to teach class, I think of my one word; when I'm uninspired by my life, I think of my one word; when I'm reluctant to reach out to someone, I think of my one word; when I'm planning my future, I think of my one word—my one word motivates, inspires, drives, and guides me. Following my one word is an emotional "diet" plan that keeps me healthy. Being led by my one word makes me feel hopeful and free and allows me to drop the weight of life. My one word is a compass that allows my spirit to manifest into anything I want it to.

After all, it's my one word that led me to *connect* to you.

My parents' individual lessons in happiness and balance have allowed me to fully *connect* to my mind, body, heart, and spirit; their mutual lesson in the constancy of change has enabled me to *connect* the path of my life; and my desire to *connect* is the reason I am a teacher and is the purpose of this book.

I hope you feel inspired to connect to your one and find your true self. Consider communicating and interpreting your own life lessons, saying "thank you" to your parents, and discovering your one word. It may not happen immediately or easily but if it eventually does, I hope that my experiences, choices, life lessons, and words have helped you.

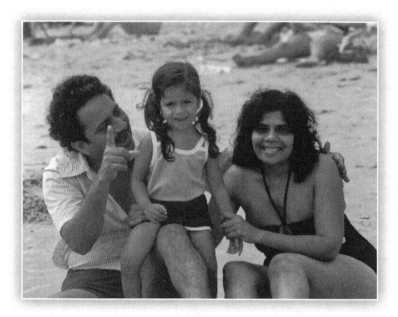

If finding the incentive to start the journey of thanking your parents is difficult, take a moment, clear your mind, and think about a few words, ideas, or lessons that your parents taught you. Consider how they shaped you both negatively and positively. You may be surprised at the result and how it motivates you.

Solution, problem, success, failure, shut up, sit, smile, love, be, treat, let go, live, love, thank you, *happiness*, *balance* and *connect*—Words DO matter.

What's your one word? If you don't know your one word, are you on the path to discovering it? If you know your one word, are you living it?

Find your word. Let it be your true self. Live it every day. Share it with others.

CONNECT TO YOUR ONE

I would love to connect with you beyond this book. My websites, www.nalinikids.org and www.nalinimethod.com are places for you to connect and join others on their path to their one word.

Thanks for helping me *connect.*

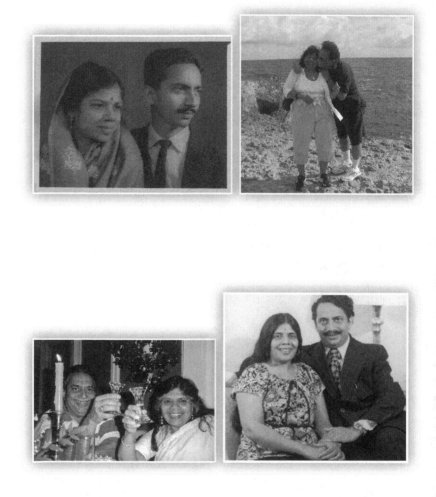

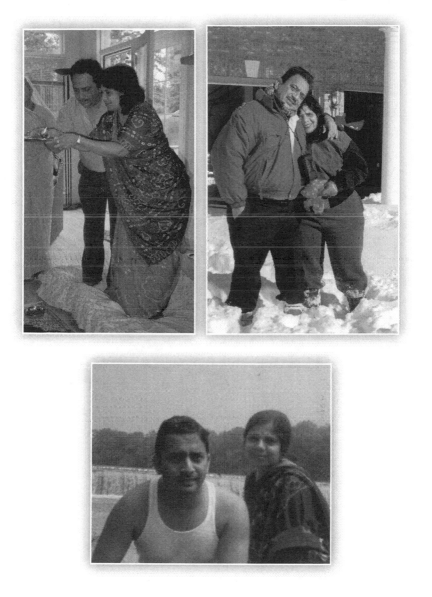

Made in the USA
Middletown, DE
22 October 2015